WISHING YOU A SPEEDY RECOVERY!

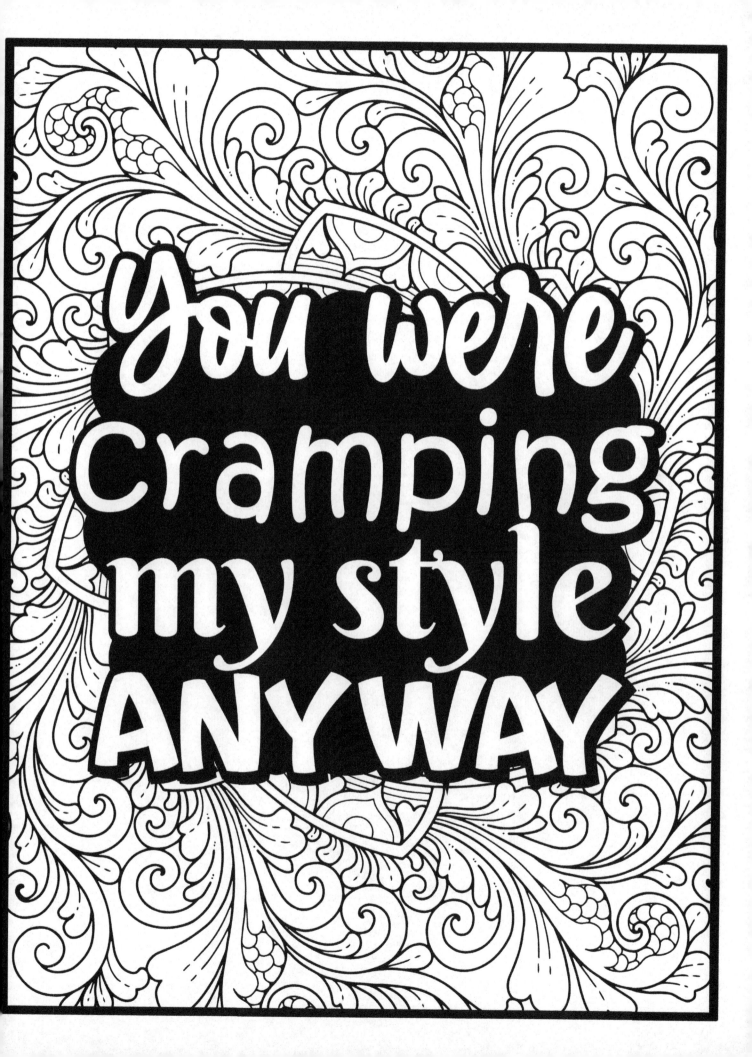

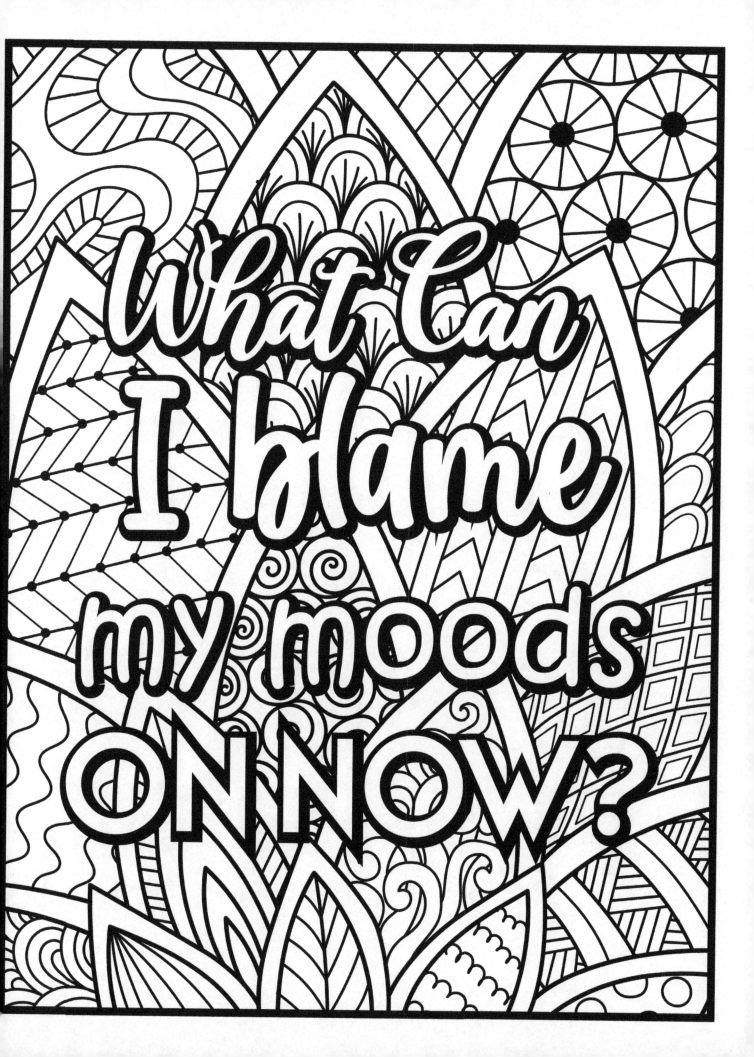

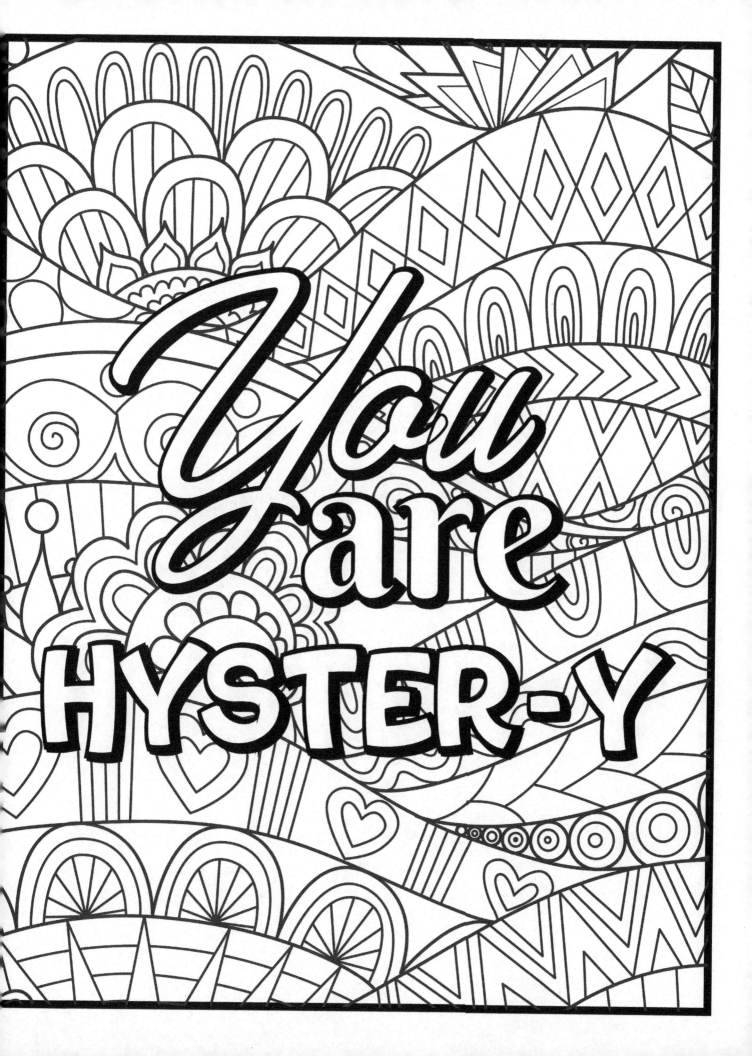

Uterus Apart 8(

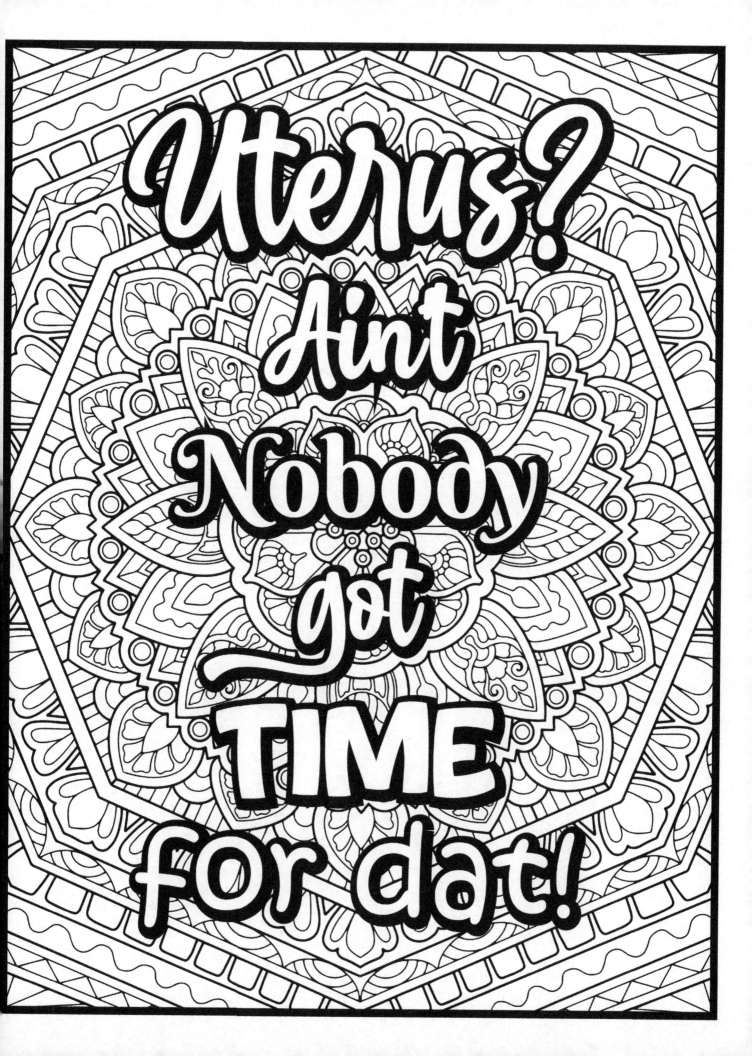

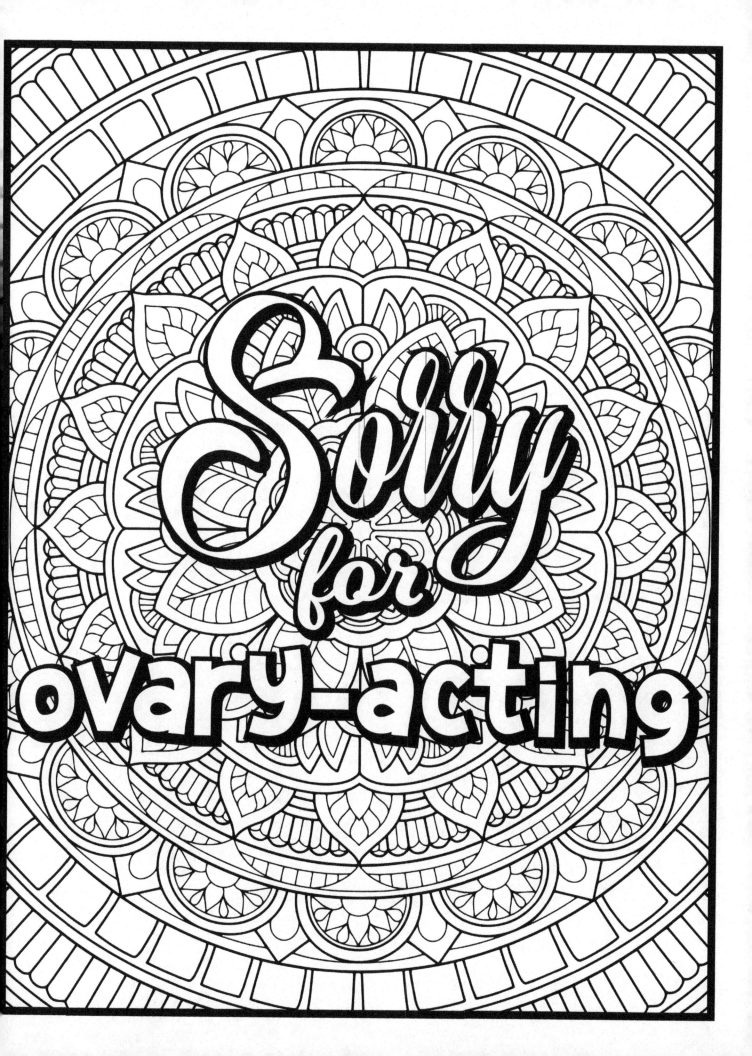

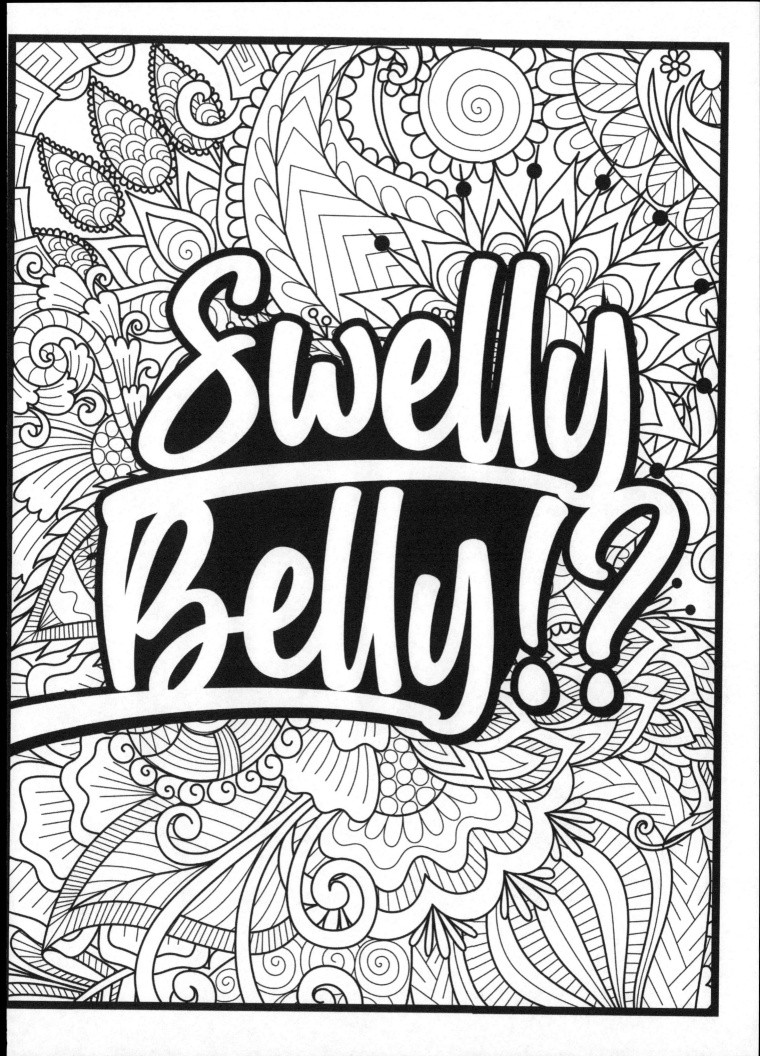

Snip
Snip
HOORAY

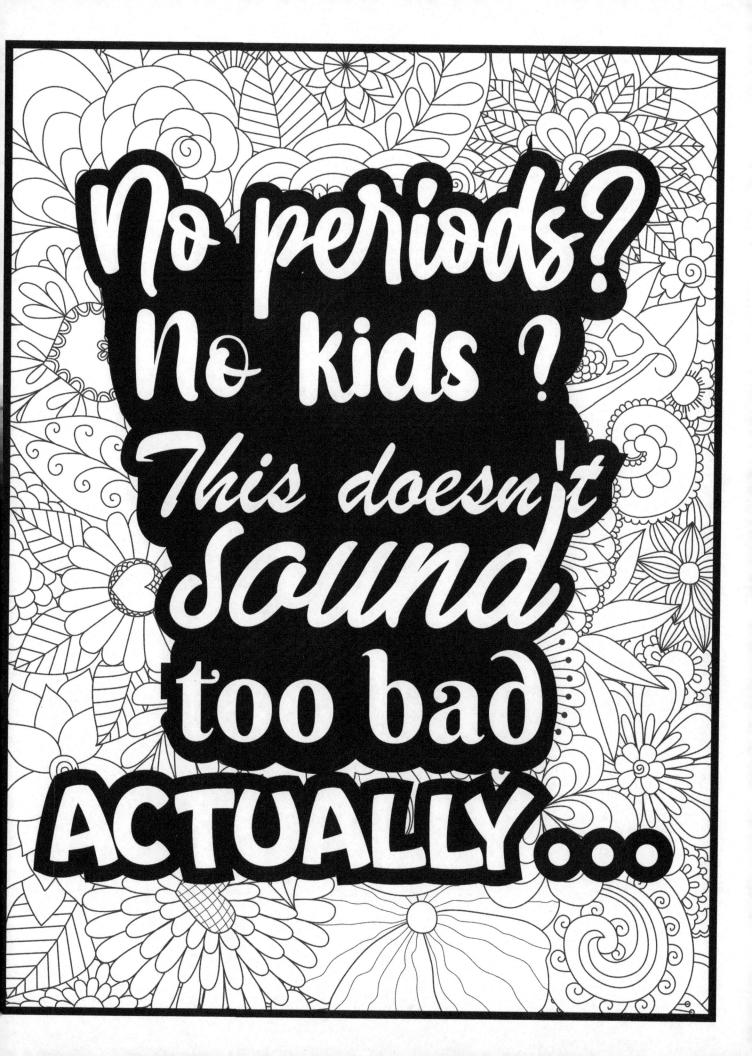

I'm NOW a hyster Sister

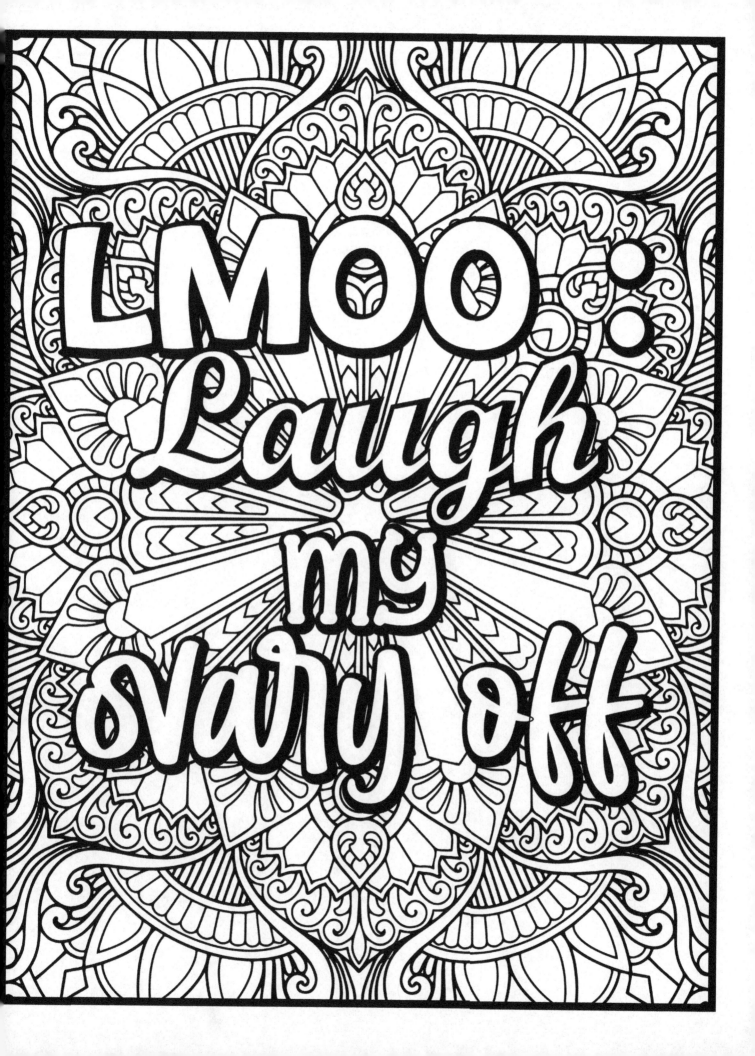

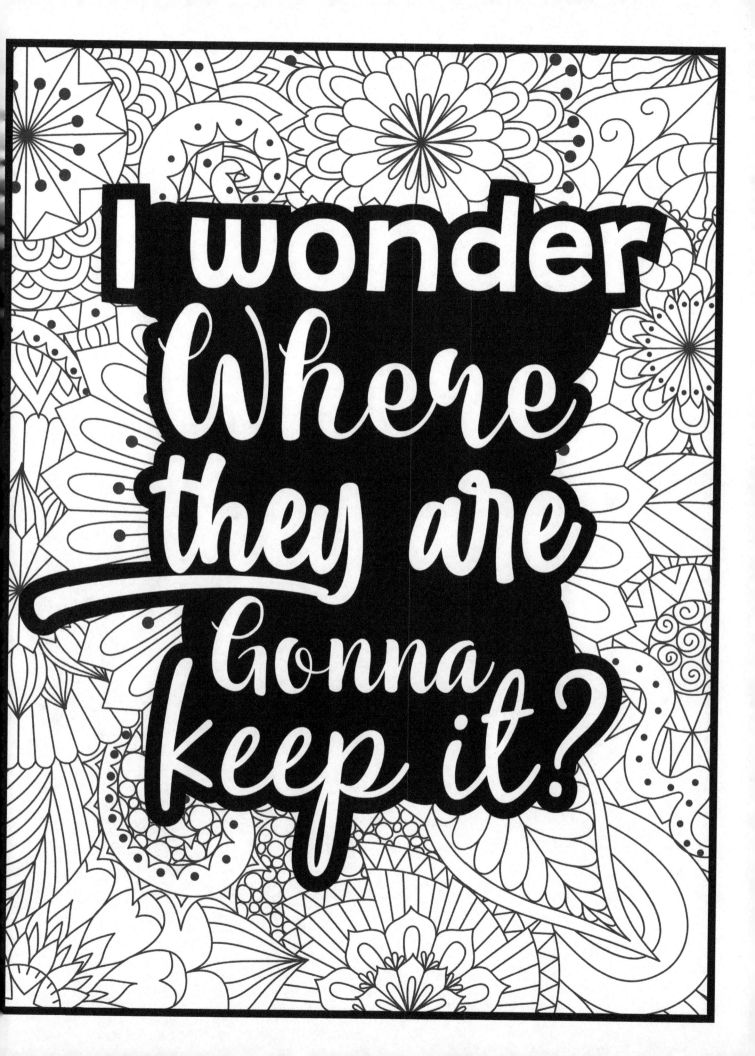

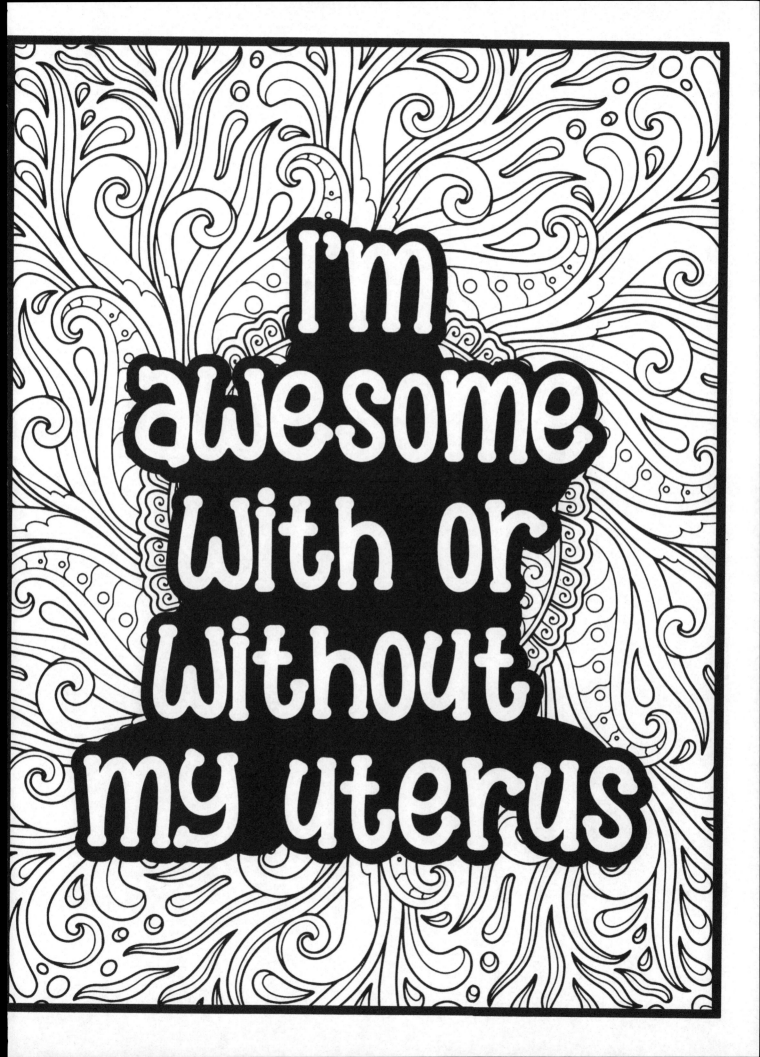

I'm awesome with or without my uterus

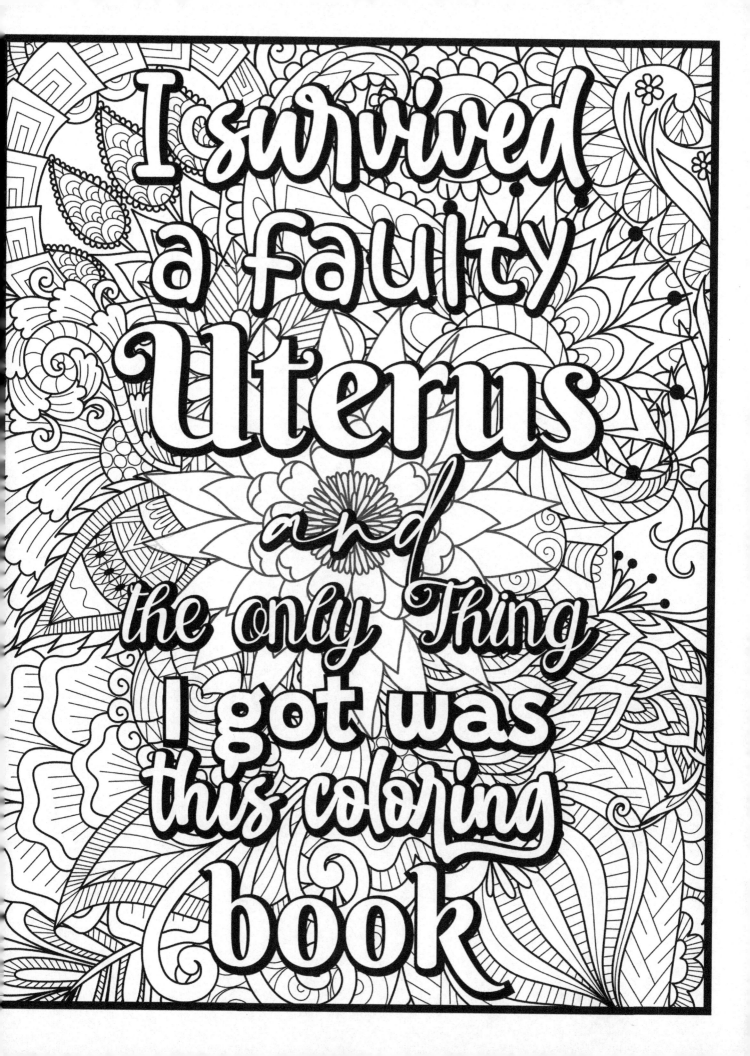

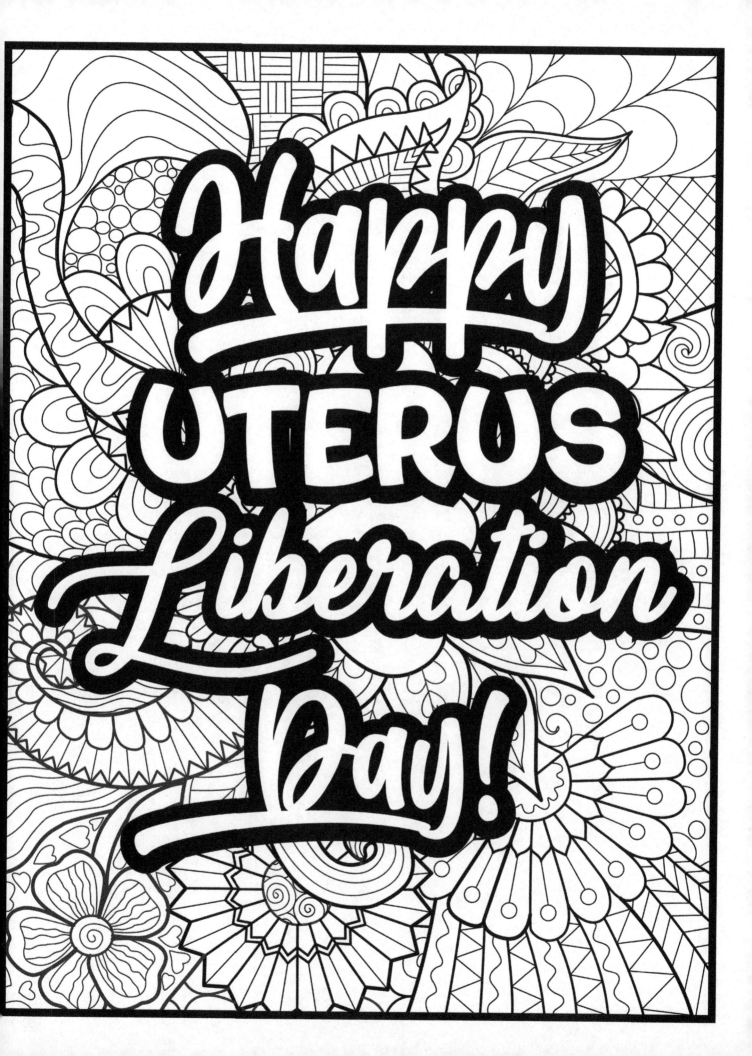

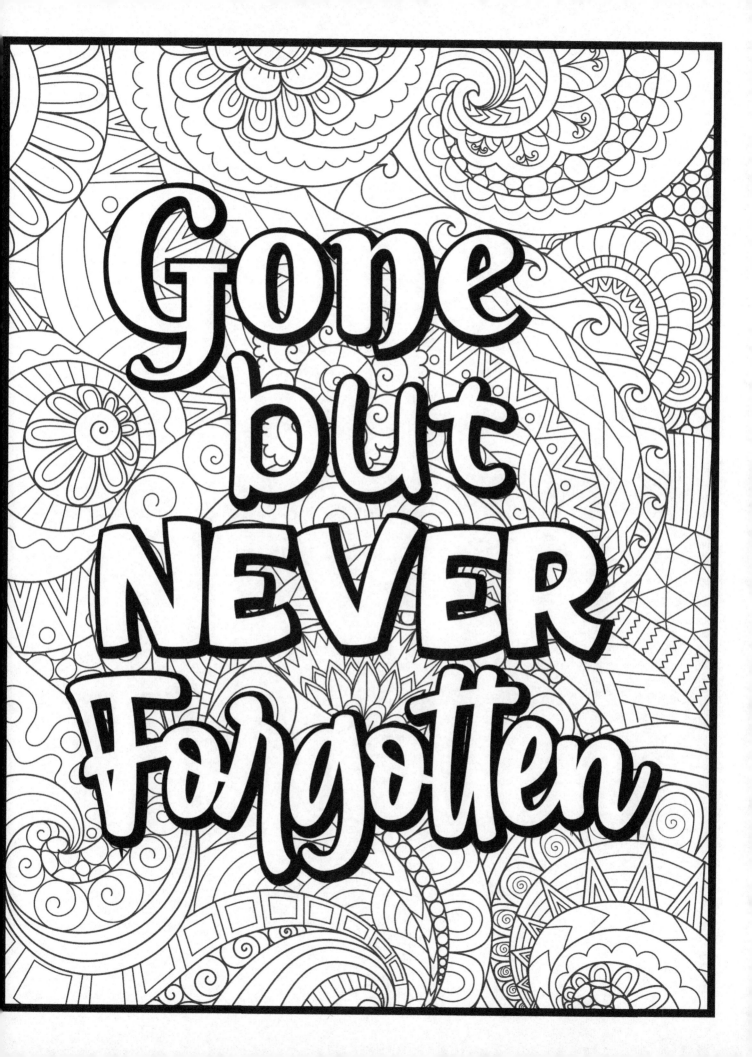

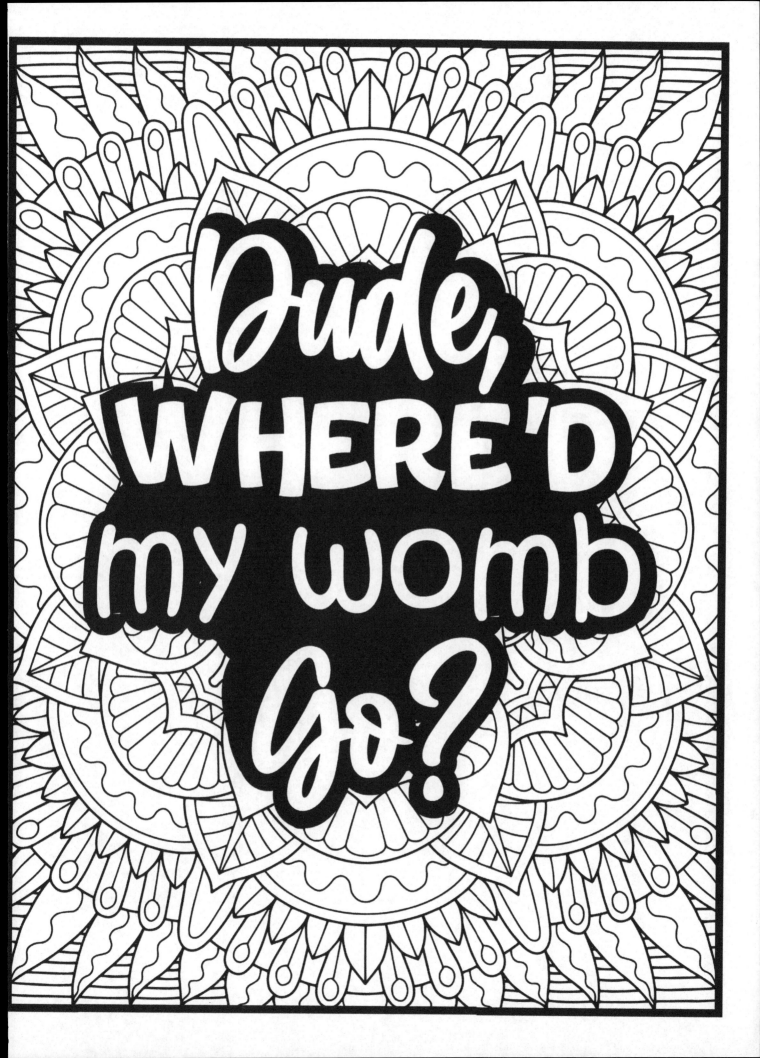

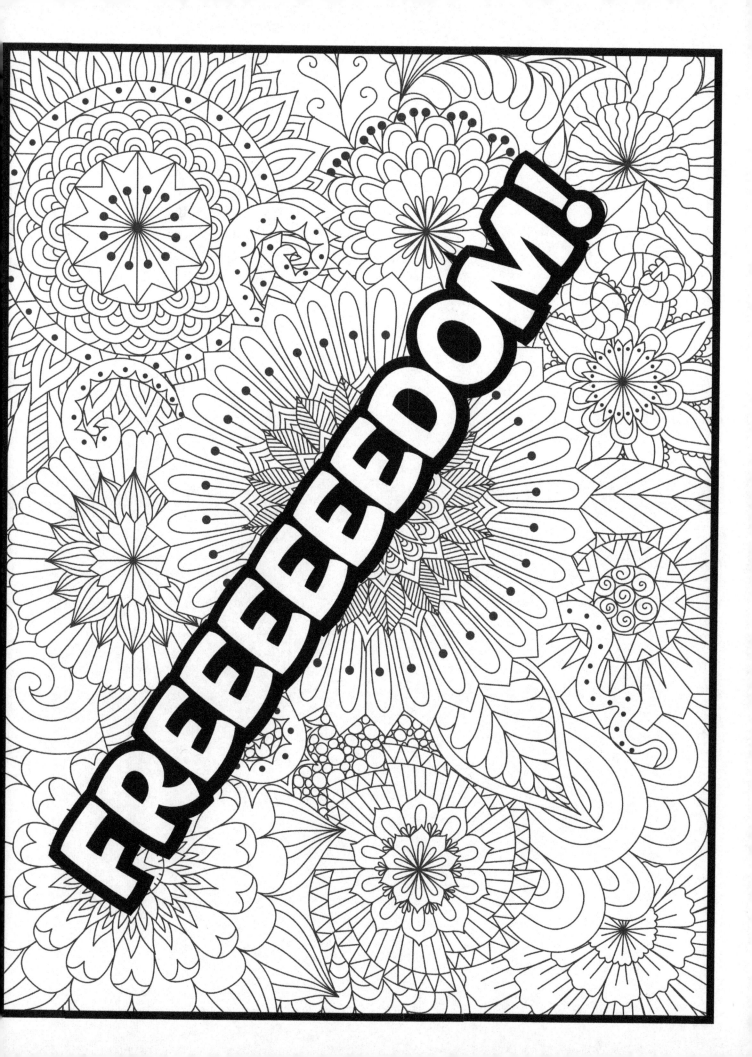

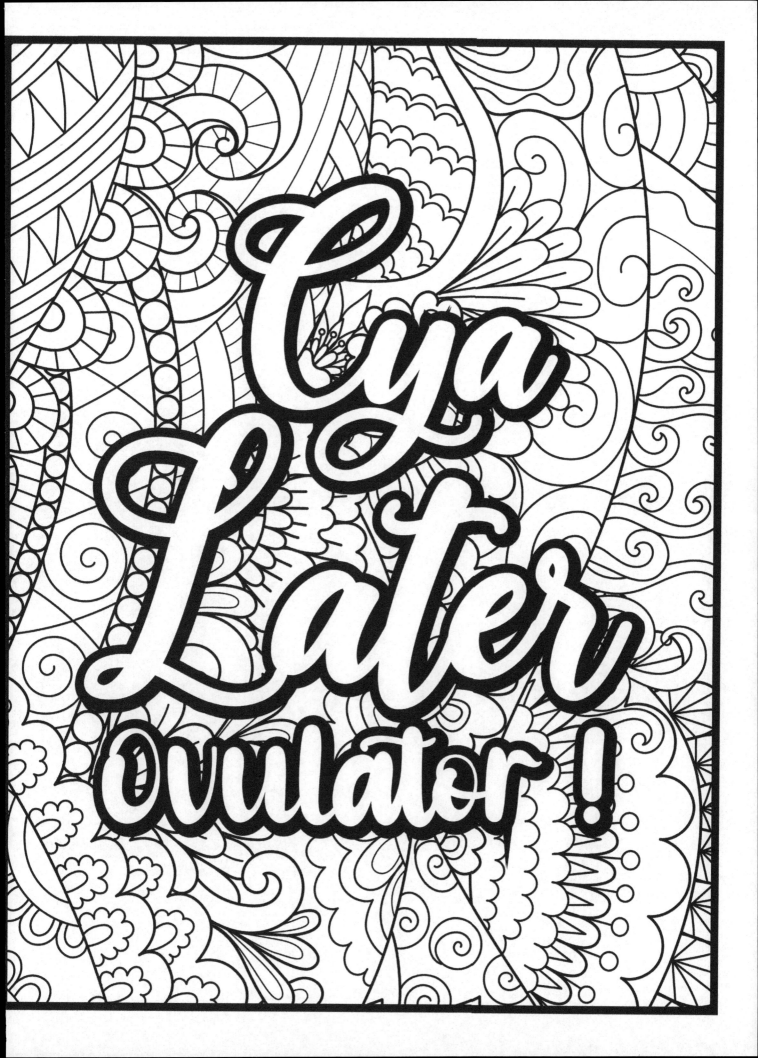

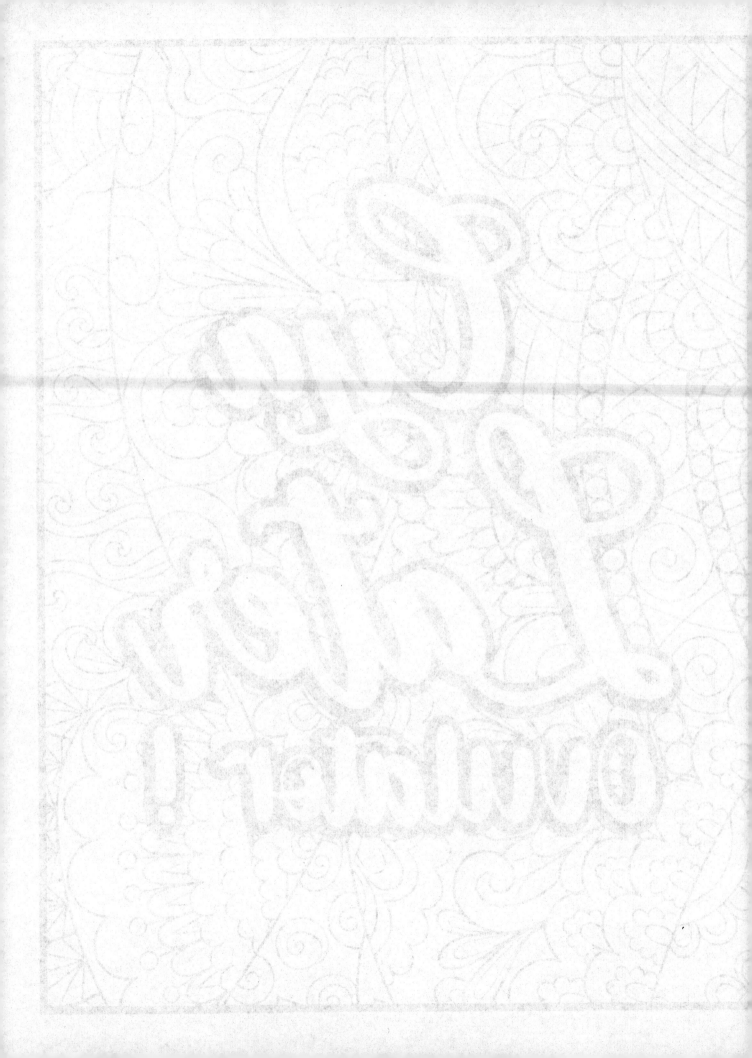

Dear Mother nature, I'd like to cancel my monthly Subscription

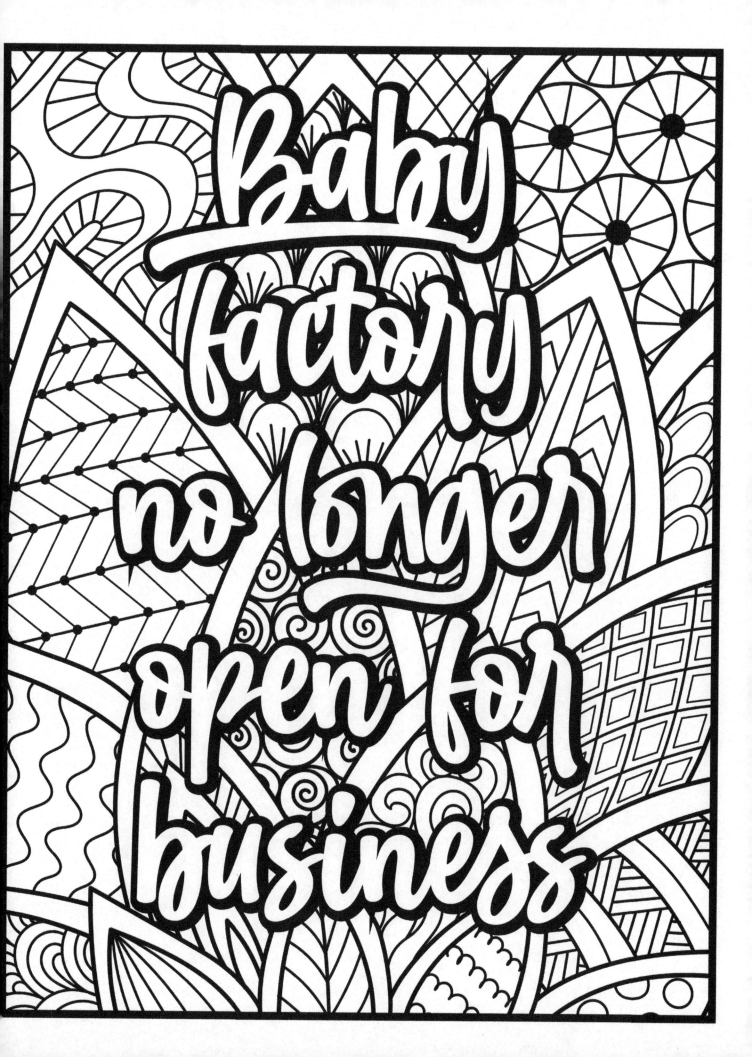

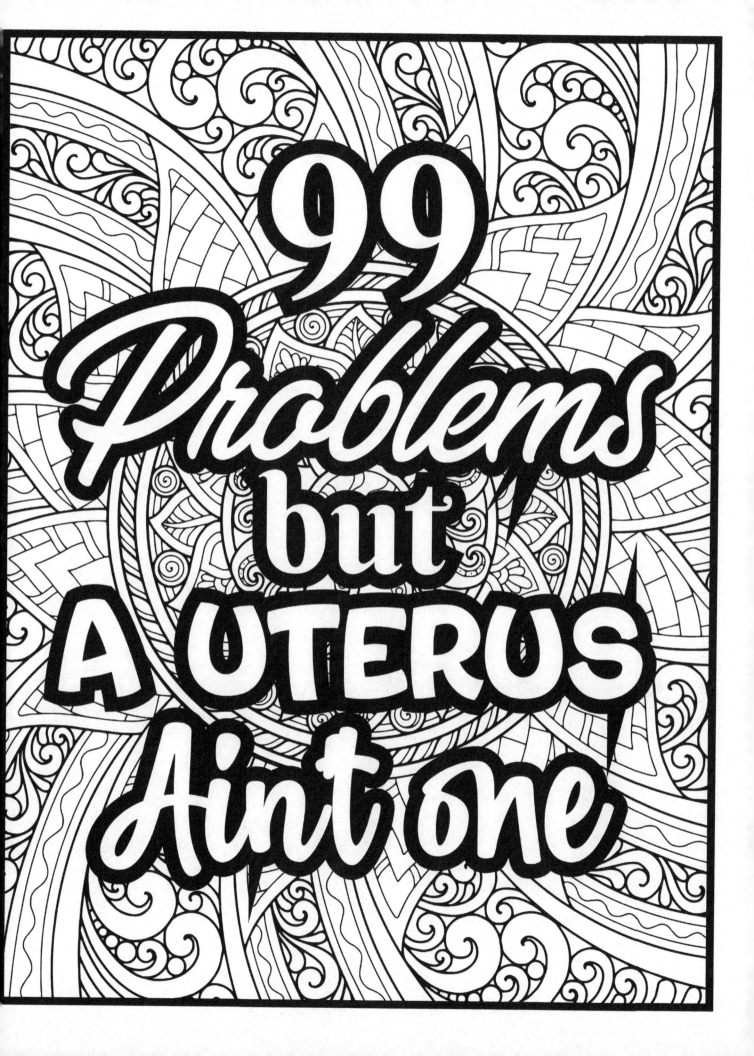

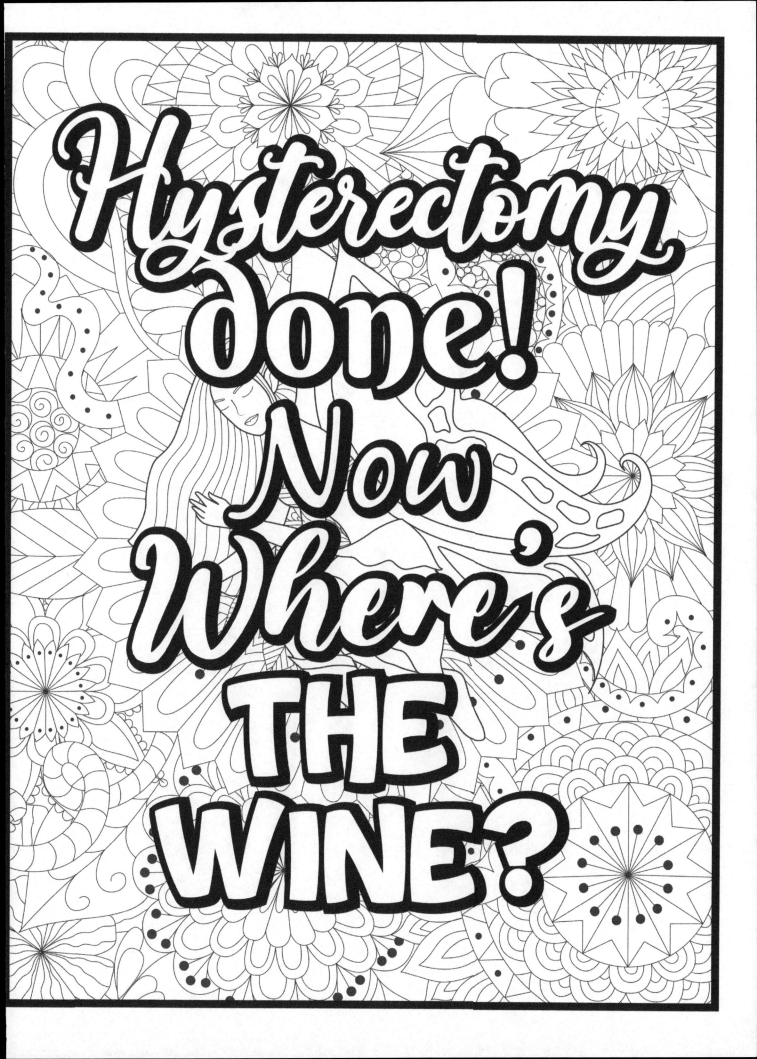

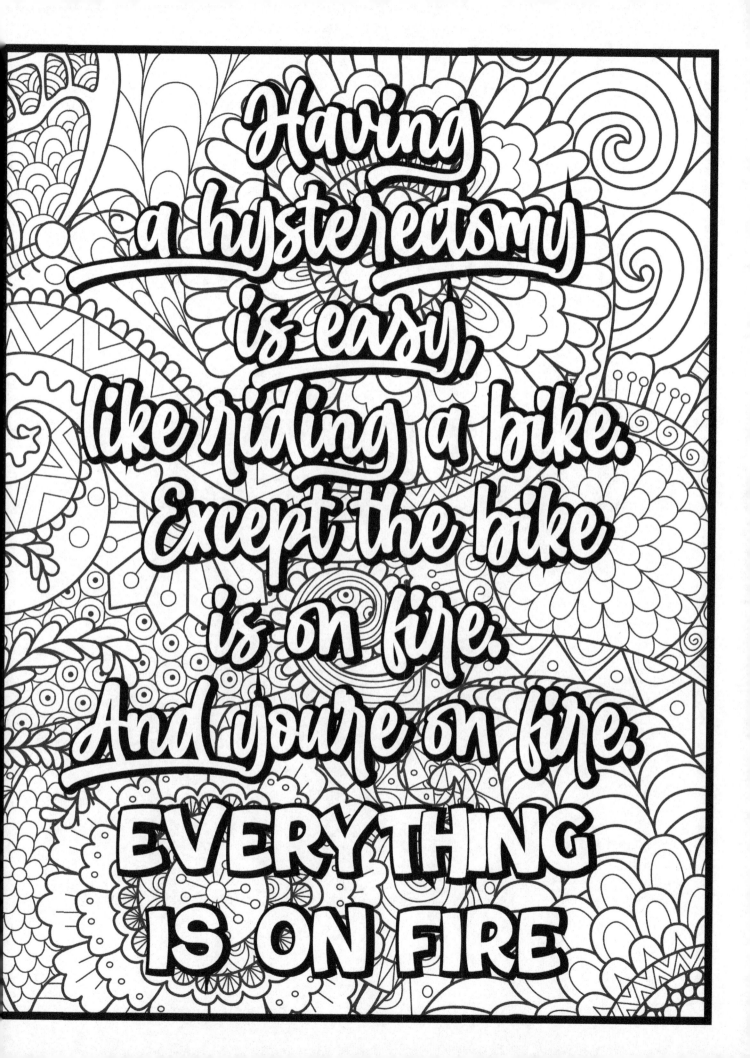

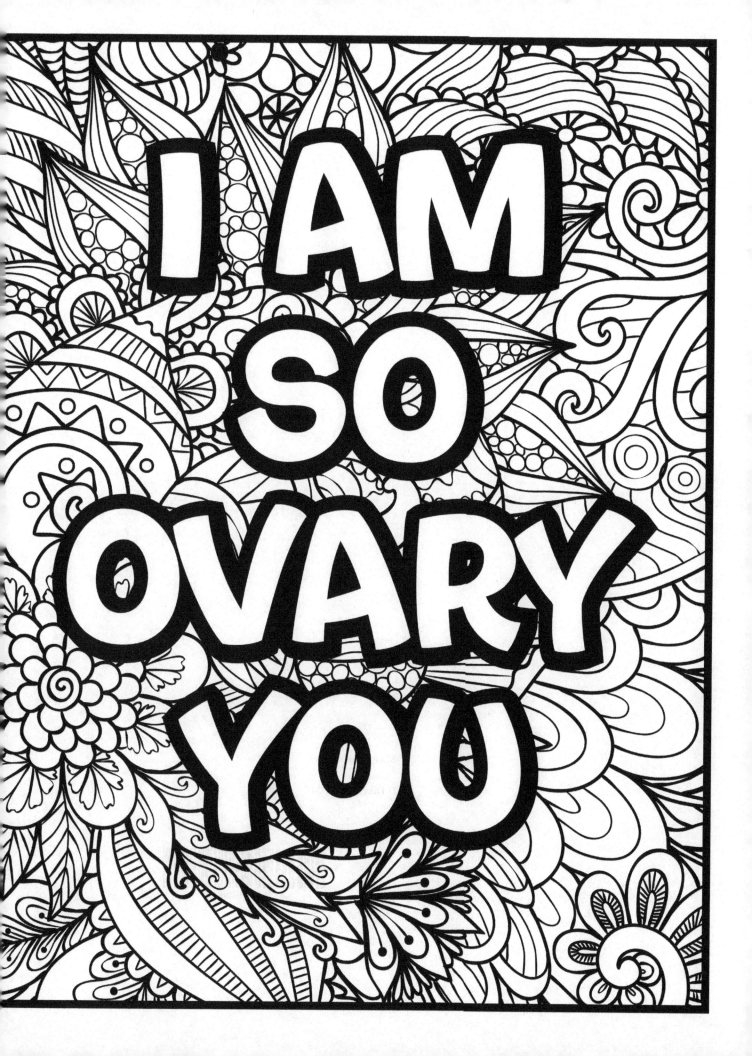

Made in the USA
Columbia, SC
03 December 2024